HSA: Start Here

S. J. Klumpenhower

HSA: Start Here

Copyright © Erisa Trust Company, Inc. All rights reserved.

No part of this publication may be reproduced, stored in a retrieval system or transmitted in any form or by any means except as permitted by law. For more information contact Erisa Trust Company, 1200 San Pedro Dr. NE, Albuquerque, NM 87110, (505) 216-7800, or online at www.erisa-trust.com.

> **Disclaimer:** Please note that this book is meant as a reference guide only and does not serve in any way as legal, tax, or financial advice. The laws surrounding this issue are regularly updating, and sections of this book are liable to change as the healthcare legislation informing this issue changes. Consult your professional legal, tax, or financial advisor for assistance.

ISBN: 9781625034328

Acknowledgements

I would like to express my gratitude to C.S. Hwa, Ph.D., founder of Erisa Trust Company, for sponsoring this project. It has been inspiring to see his strong belief in the lasting and profound impact of HSA legislation on the way healthcare will be managed by and for the American public.

Additional thanks to the following individuals, who helped to bring this book to production:

Legal Advisor: Larry Grudzien   Cover Design: Xiaoxia Li
Copy Editor: Danny Saldaña   Formatting: Susannah Davenport

Table of Contents

Introduction: What is an HSA? i
    Why HSA? i
    Comparing Tax-Favored Accounts iii
    How to Use this Book iii
Chapter 1: Eligibility 1
    HSA-Eligible Health Plans 1
    Other Coverage 3
        Health FSAs and HRAs 5
Chapter 2: Contributions 7
    Contribution Limits 7
    Who Can Contribute 10
        Comparability and Nondiscrimination 11
        Owners and 2% or More Shareholders 12
    Scheduling Contributions 12
    Account Rollovers and Transfers 13
        HSA-Rollover 13
        IRA Transfer 14
    Excess Contributions 14
Chapter 3: Distributions 17
    Qualified Expenses 17
    The Distribution Process 19

　　　　Save Receipts 19

　　　　Fees on Non-Eligible Withdrawals............................... 20

Chapter 4: Account Management 23

　　　　Establishing Your HSA 23

　　　　Invest your Savings 24

　　　　　　　Fund HSA First.. 26

　　　　Tips on Saving 28

　　　　Tax Reporting 29

Chapter 5: What about…? 33

　　　　Medicare 33

　　　　FMLA... 33

　　　　Continuing Coverage 34

　　　　Losing and Regaining Eligibility.................................... 34

　　　　TRICARE and IHS Coverage 36

　　　　Divorce 37

　　　　Death..37

　　　　State Rules 37

Conclusion: Is HSA Right for You? 39

　　　　Taking Control of Your Health 39

Appendix I: Qualified Medical Expenses.. 43

Glossary 47

Resources... 49

Introduction: What is an HSA?

A long life of health and financial security is an important goal for all Americans, but that's often easier said than done. You likely know some steps that can improve your health and finances, like eating better, exercising more, and putting money into savings. But did you know that switching your health plan can also help you save for the future? Switching plans can also help you to develop a pattern of better living so you can live a healthier life.

An alternative to a traditional healthcare plan is a Health Savings Account (HSA) matched with an eligible High-Deductible Health Plan (HDHP). This health plan is designed to give you more control over your health spending and help you save money for the future.

> **Health Savings Account** – an account where you save money for your healthcare expenses. It is owned by a single person and maintained by an IRS-approved trust company or custodian.

Money that goes into an HSA is yours. You can use it when you need it, the funds roll over from year to year, and the account will stay with you even if you change jobs. Plus, money that goes into an HSA is tax-free or tax deductible, money you make from investing your HSA dollars accumulates tax-free, and any money spent on qualified medical expenses is tax-free: the triple-tax advantage.

Why HSA?

Medical expenses in America have been on the rise for decades now. In 1970, the average cost spent on healthcare per person was $327 a year (about $2,150 after inflation), and healthcare costs made up 6.2% of all spending in America. In 2016, the average amount spent on healthcare per person was $9,892—four times the 1970 average. This means that in 2016, Americans spent a total of $3.3 trillion on healthcare, making up 17.2% of all spending in America. [i]

In comparison, education made up only 6.2% of all spending in America, [ii] and military costs only accounted for 3.3%. [iii] And our healthcare expenses will only keep growing.

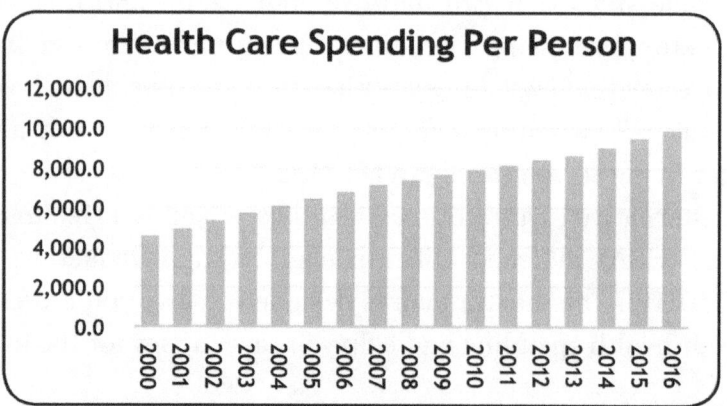

So how can we try to limit healthcare costs? Many people believe that one of the best ways is to give more control over healthcare spending back to the consumer: you.

Consumer-Driven Health Plans (CDHPs), also known as high-deductible health plans (HDHPs), are designed to give you more control over your spending and make you more aware of the cost of your medical care. When you are more aware of your healthcare costs, you're more likely to look at your options and choose the best care. This also encourages healthcare providers to offer better prices and reduces costs for everyone.

Based on this theory, HDHPs and their attached HSAs were established under the 2003 Medicare Prescription Drug, Improvement, and Modernization Act. Since then, enrollment in HSAs has risen to over 22 million people as of 2017. Experts estimate that people will deposit $44 billion to their HSAs in 2018 alone. [iv]

Comparing Tax-Favored Accounts

An HSA has advantages over other medical spending accounts like a Health Flexible Spending Account (Health FSA) or Health Reimbursement Arrangement (HRA). FSAs are "use-it-or-lose-it" accounts that expire at the end of the coverage period or at the end of the grace or carryover period, if applicable. HRA funds may also expire at the end of the coverage period or carry over, depending on the arrangement the employer has set up. Additionally, both FSAs and HRAs are tied to your job, so if you lose your job you also lose your account and can only reimburse qualified expenses from when you were employed or continuing your coverage through COBRA. But your HSA money never expires and will stay with you no matter your employment status.

HSAs even have advantages over retirement investment accounts like your 401(k) or IRA. Money that goes into one of these funds is taxed either when the money goes in or when it comes out. IRAs also require that you start withdrawing money in the year you turn age 70½. There is no requirement to withdraw your HSA money at any point, and you can make tax-free or tax-deductible contributions and tax-free withdrawals for eligible medical expenses no matter when you request a reimbursement.

	Health FSA	HRA	IRA	Roth IRA	HSA
Tax-Free Contributions	✓	✓	✓		✓
Tax-Free Distributions	✓	✓		✓	✓
Tax-Free Investments			✓	✓	✓
Account moves with you			✓	✓	✓
Money doesn't expire			✓	✓	✓

How to Use this Book

This book is divided into chapters based on the different parts of owning an HSA, starting with determining eligibility and walking through how to make contributions, request distributions, and manage your account. The last chapter deals with specific scenarios that might affect you. In the back, you'll find a list with some of the qualified medical expenses that you can use your HSA money for as well as a glossary of useful terms and resources for further research.

You can choose to read the book straight through, or you can skip to a particular chapter if you have questions about something specific. While the book is designed to build on itself as you go through, each section does stand alone and can be read separately. Feel free to take things at your own pace and reference items as needed.

Chapter 1: Eligibility

A Health Savings Account (HSA) is an account for you to save money for your qualified medical expenses. You own the money in your HSA, and once money is contributed to your account you can access it whenever you need.

Establishing an HSA requires a little more than just putting some money in a jar and claiming it on your taxes, though. Only eligible individuals can establish an HSA, and only with an IRS-approved custodian or administrator.

Eligibility is determined on the first day of each month and lasts for the entire month. If you become eligible in the middle of a month, you'll need to wait until the next month to establish your HSA. To be eligible, you must be:

1) Covered by an HSA-eligible health plan,
2) Not covered by any disqualifying medical coverage,
3) Not receiving Medicare benefits, and
4) Not claimable as a dependent on anyone else's taxes.

You can be eligible if you are covered under your own HSA-eligible health plan, your spouse's plan, or, in some cases, your parents' plan. Each account is based on an individual person's eligibility, and each person has their own HSA that belongs only to them. Family HSAs or shared HSAs do not exist. However, if you have an HSA, you can use it to reimburse your own, your spouse's, and your tax dependents' qualified medical expenses. Your spouse can also start their own HSA as long as they are eligible.

HSA-Eligible Health Plans

The major difference between a traditional health plan and an HSA-eligible high-deductible health plan is in the name: "high deductible." In insurance, the deductible is the amount that you need to pay before the insurance company (or employer, in the case of a self-funded health plan) will help to pay for qualified expenses. Anything you pay before you meet your deductible will be your responsibility, with no co-pays.

The IRS sets limits every year on the minimum deductible a plan must have to be considered HSA-eligible. For 2018 and 2019, the minimum deductible for an individual is $1,350 and the family minimum is $2,700.

Some plans have an embedded deductible for their family plans where the deductible is lower for each individual person than for the whole family amount. For example, the family deductible might be $3,000, which would qualify the plan for HSA eligibility. But if it has an embedded deductible at $1,500 per person, that amount is lower than the family minimum and means the health plan is not HSA-eligible.

	2018	2019
Minimum Deductible	Self only: $1,350	Self only: $1,350
	Family: $2,700	Family: $2,700
Maximum Out of Pocket	Self only: $6,650	Self only: $6,750
	Family: $13,300	Family: $13,500

The other thing an HSA-eligible plan must include is an out-of-pocket maximum, which is also set by the IRS. There is a limit on how much money you pay out of pocket before your insurance starts paying for everything, including deductibles, copayments, and coinsurance. This protects you against sudden emergency expenses that leave you without any remaining savings. The out-of-pocket maximum only applies to in-network coverage; out of network coverage can have a limit higher than the IRS statute.

If a plan doesn't have both a minimum deductible at or above the limit and an out-of-pocket maximum at or below the limit, then it doesn't qualify as an HSA-eligible health plan. These limits change annually, so most insurance companies and employers will adjust their high-deductible health plans as needed to maintain HSA-eligibility.

Anything between the deductible and the out-of-pocket maximum is covered by coinsurance. You'll pay part of the cost, usually somewhere

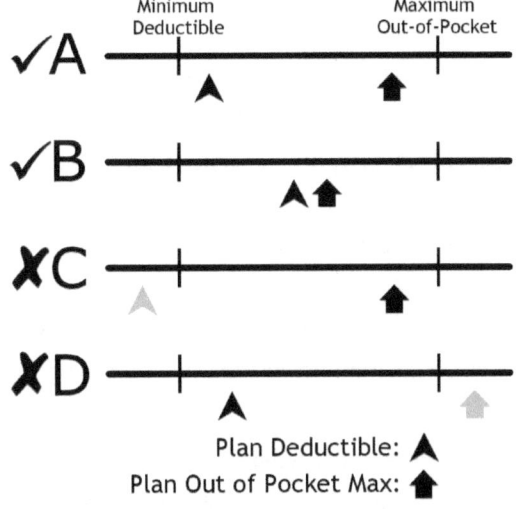

between 5% and 20%, and your insurance will cover the rest.

Traditional health plans also have a deductible, but it is generally much lower. The trade-off is that high-deductible health plans usually have lower premiums, so that you don't pay as much out of your paycheck. The money you save on premiums can then be put into your HSA and used for current or future health care expenses.

While an HSA-eligible health plan doesn't offer you a low copay at the doctor's office, it will usually negotiate better prices for you within a network of doctors. It will also cover you for preventive care, including regular check-ups and specific medicines.

Other Coverage

In addition to being enrolled in an HSA-eligible health plan, you also need to make sure that you aren't enrolled in any disqualifying coverage. Common types of disqualifying coverage include:
- Medicare
- A spouse or parent's health insurance or other health coverage
- Health FSAs/HRAs (yours or your spouse's)

Accident, disability, long-term, and property insurance will not impact your HSA eligibility. You are also allowed to have insurance for a specific disease and tort insurance that provides a set amount of money for specific situations like hospitalization. A discount card for prescriptions is allowed, since you aren't being reimbursed for any costs.

Eligibility Example 1

Alex's workplace has just started offering an HSA-eligible health plan. He and his wife Barbara decide to switch from a traditional health plan to the HSA-eligible health plan. They have no other disqualifying coverage, so both Alex and Barbara are eligible to establish their HSAs on the first day of the month following their switch.

Eligibility Example 2

Abigail and her husband Ben are interested in signing up for HSAs. Ben has individual coverage on a traditional health plan through his workplace. Abigail has an HSA-eligible plan that covers herself, Ben, and their two children, Candice and Daniel. Candice is 25 and works full time, and Daniel is 19 and attending college.

Abigail is eligible to establish an HSA, since she isn't under any disqualifying coverage, but Ben is not because of his insurance through his workplace. Ben's qualified medical expenses that aren't covered by his insurance can still be reimbursed from Abigail's HSA.

Candice is old enough that she is no longer able to be claimed as a dependent on her parents' taxes, even though she is on their health plan. She cannot be reimbursed from Abigail's HSA, but she can open her own HSA. Daniel is still a tax dependent, so he can't establish his own HSA. His qualified medical expenses can be reimbursed from Abigail's HSA.

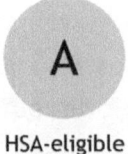
HSA-eligible
Can Reimburse:
A, B, D

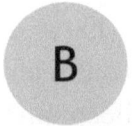
Not HSA-eligible

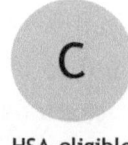
HSA-eligible
Can Reimburse:
C

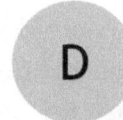
Not HSA-eligible

Health FSAs and HRAs

If you or your spouse participate in a Health Flexible Spending Account (Health FSA) or Health Reimbursement Arrangement (HRA) when you join an HSA-eligible health plan, you will have to wait to establish an HSA until your Health FSA or HRA closes at the end of the plan year. Because your Health FSA and HRA money can be used for your medical expenses as well as your spouse and dependents, it makes everyone ineligible to establish and contribute to an HSA.

Making the switch from a Health FSA or HRA to an HSA can get tricky, since some FSA and HRA programs have a grace or carryover period that will cover you into the next year if you still have money in your account. The way to avoid this is to make sure that all the money in your FSA is spent before the new year so that nothing carries over. Otherwise, you will have to wait until the end of the grace period to establish your HSA.

Some FSAs and HRAs don't count as disqualifying coverage. These Limited Purpose plans (LPFSAs and LPHRAs) might only cover dental, vision, or preventive expenses, or only pay for medical expenses after the deductible has been met. Because these don't reimburse medical expenses before the deductible is met, they can work with your HSA instead of making you ineligible. A non-healthcare FSA, such as dependent care or transit, will also not impact your HSA eligibility.

Eligibility Example 3

Audrey and her husband Brent are both covered under Audrey's HSA-eligible health plan, and both have HSAs. Brent's workplace just started offering a Health FSA option that Brent would like to sign up for. Audrey asks him to check to see if it's a limited purpose FSA before he signs up.

Brent is so excited about the FSA option that he signs up without checking to see if it is an LPFSA. It is not a limited purpose account, and now he and Audrey are both ineligible to contribute for the entire year he has his general purpose Health

FSA. They can start contributing to their HSAs the following year so long as they don't still have money in the Health FSA account that might roll over into a grace period. Otherwise, they will have to wait until the end of the grace period to be eligible.

Chapter 2: Contributions

Contribution Limits

Just like there are limits on your deductible and out-of-pocket maximum, there is a limit on how much money can be contributed to your HSA each year. This amount is also set each year by the IRS and is generally increased to account for inflation. There is also a catch-up contribution for people who are 55 years old or above that is applied in addition to the regular contribution.

	2018	2019
Individual Limit	$3,450	$3,500
Family Limit	$6,900	$7,000
Catch-up Contribution	$1,000	$1,000

Your contribution limit is based on what level of HSA-eligible plan you are enrolled in. If you are enrolled in a family health plan that covers you and at least one other person, you are eligible to make contributions up to the family limit. This is true even if no one else in your family is eligible for their own HSA. If you are enrolled in a self-only HSA-eligible health plan, you can only contribute up to the individual limit, even if you are married or have children.

A catch-up contribution of $1,000 is available to anyone who is 55 years or older by year's end. This contribution is only available to the person who is over 55, so if you are 53 and your spouse is 56, they are eligible to make a catch-up contribution to their HSA, but the money can't go into yours. However, as long as you are HSA-eligible for the whole year, you are eligible for the entire catch-up contribution, no matter when in the year you turn age 55.

> **Contribution Example 1**
>
> Both Andrew and his wife Beverly are eligible to establish and contribute to an HSA under the same family coverage HSA-eligible plan. Andrew is 52, and Beverly just turned 55. They can choose to split their total limit for a contribution however they'd like between the two accounts. Andrew and Beverly decide to split the amount in half for 2018, with Andrew contributing $3,450 to his account. Because Beverly has turned 55, she can contribute an extra $1,000 to her account, bringing her total to $4,450.
>
> This extra catch-up contribution can only go to Beverly's HSA, even if they were to split their family contribution differently. So they could choose to put all $6,900 of the regular contribution into Andrew's account, but the $1,000 catch-up contribution would still have to go to Beverly's account.

If you and your spouse both are HSA-eligible, your total contributions added together can't be more than the family contribution limit for the year. This rule is specifically for spouses; as of this publication, if your domestic partner or children are HSA-eligible under a family health plan, they can contribute the full family amount to their HAS without impacting your contribution limit.

Remember that each HSA is owned by an individual person. There are no family HSAs that are shared by everyone, but a person with an account can reimburse their own, their spouse's, and their tax dependents' qualified expenses.

> **Contribution Example 2**
>
> Alice is 24 years old and works full-time. She is still covered under her parents' HSA-eligible health plan, and since she is not considered a tax dependent she is eligible to open her own HSA. Because she is covered under a family health plan, even though it is not her own plan, she can contribute up

> to the family limit for the year. She contributes a full $6,900 to her HSA. This amount does not count toward her parents' contribution limit.

The contribution limit is a yearly amount, and if you are only eligible part of the year then you are only eligible to make a partial contribution based on the number of months you were eligible. To find out how much you are allowed to contribute, you will have to prorate your contribution. Take the yearly limit and divide by 12, then multiply that by the number of months you were eligible. Prorating also applies to the catch-up contribution.

> **Yearly Amount ÷ 12 × Months Eligible = Limit**

The exception to prorating your contribution is called the Last Month Rule. If you are eligible to establish an HSA on December 1st of any year, you can choose to make a full annual contribution, even if you weren't eligible for the whole year. If you decide to do this, you will need to stay eligible for the entire next year: a 12-consecutive-month testing period. If you lose your eligibility at any time during this testing period, you will have to go back and prorate your contribution based on the usual rules. Any extra money you contributed will need to be taken out of your HSA, counted as part of your income on your next round of taxes, and both income tax and an excise tax of 10% on the amount paid.

> ***Contribution Example 3***
> Adam gets a new job April 13, 2018. He enrolls in an HSA-eligible health plan with individual coverage and is HSA-eligible as of May 1, 2018. He establishes his account immediately and feels very confident about his new job and health plan, so he contributes all the way up to his individual limit for the year as soon as he can using the last-month rule.

On August 5, Adam marries Beth and decides to use the last-month rule again to contribute all the way up to the family limit for 2018. By the end of the year, he contributes the full $6,900 into his HSA.

Unfortunately, things start going downhill for Adam in 2019. His marriage to Beth falls apart, and he gets divorced in June of 2019, meaning he's failed the test period for his family coverage. He calculates his allowable contribution for 2018 with 4 months of family coverage (starting September 1) and the rest at individual coverage. This comes to $2,300 in family coverage plus $2,300 in individual coverage, totaling $4,600. He plans to count the remaining $2,300 he contributed in 2018 as income on his next year's taxes and pay regular taxes and the additional 10% tax.

Then, in October 2019, Adam loses his job. He chooses not to continue his coverage through COBRA, so he fails the testing period for individual coverage as well. His new contribution limit for 2018 is $3,450, and he will have to claim $3,450 on his income taxes and pay the 10% excise tax.

Who Can Contribute

You can add money to your HSA. So can your employer. So can your grandmother, or your best friend, or just about anyone. As long as you are eligible to make contributions, it doesn't matter what the source of those contributions is. And once the money is in your account, it is yours, all without you paying any taxes on the amount.

No matter who the money came from, the tax break is only for the person who received the money. So if your Great-Aunt Helga puts $500 into your HSA for your birthday, you can note that contribution as a line-item deduction on your end-of-year tax return, but she cannot.

Many employers sponsor cafeteria plans, also known as Section 125 plans, where you can pick and choose which benefits you would like to enroll in and have the amount deducted pre-tax from your paycheck. This also works for HSAs, so if you have a cafeteria plan you and your employer can make pre-tax contributions to your account directly out of your paycheck. Any contributions made after taxes can be taken as a line-item deduction on your tax return in April. Be sure not to count the deduction twice, though. If the money was added pre-tax, you can't count it again as a line-item deduction.

All of these contributions from you, your employer, and your friends and relatives count toward your contribution limit. So if you contribute $1,500 and receive $1,500 from your employer, then add that $500 from Great-Aunt Helga, your total contribution is $3,500—which is above the limit for individual contributions in 2018. That's why it's important to keep track of your HSA and make sure that you aren't receiving contributions that are putting you over your contribution limit for the year.

Your contribution limit doesn't change no matter how many HSAs you have. Whether you have one account that all your money goes into or fifteen accounts that you use for different things, all the money you contributed added together can't be more than your contribution limit.

Comparability and Nondiscrimination

Employers who choose to make contributions to their employee's HSAs must make sure that the money is not being distributed unfairly. Comparability laws state that everyone within a category (full-time or part-time employee; individual, self-plus-one, self-plus-two, or self-plus-three-or-more must be offered the same amount or percentage of their pay as everyone else in their category. The only exception is that employees who are not considered to be highly compensated are allowed to receive more HSA contributions than employees who are highly compensated.

If your employer offers a cafeteria plan, which allows employees to pick and choose benefits like HSA for a pre-tax deduction, they are not required to follow comparability laws. They do, however, have to meet nondiscrimination standards as outlined in the Section 125 cafeteria plan rules. These rules are also in place to make sure that highly-compensated individuals don't get extra benefits over those who receive less pay.

Plans are tested annually to make sure they meet all the required standards for nondiscrimination and comparability.

Owners and 2% or More Shareholders

If you own your business or own more than 2% of shares in an S corporation, you cannot make pre-tax deductions to your HSA directly from your paycheck. Instead, you'll need to make your deductions post-tax and take your tax deduction as a line-item on your tax return. If you receive employer contributions directly from the company, they will be included in your income.

Scheduling Contributions

One of the benefits of an HSA is that you can adjust how much you contribute throughout the year. A Health FSA, by contrast, takes a set amount that can't be changed outside a qualifying event. With an HSA, you can choose to space your contributions evenly, to add more at the start of the year so you're more prepared for upcoming medical expenses, or to wait until the end of the year and know all your expenses. You can contribute all the way up until your tax filing deadline—usually April 15th of the following year. Just make sure your administrator knows if you are contributing money for a prior year.

You can even change your contribution schedule in the middle of the year as needed. If you are adding money after taxes, you decide when to make those contributions, to increase them, or to stop contributing completely. For money being contributed pre-tax, you are legally permitted to change your contribution schedule at least once per month. Check with your employer and administrator for advice on how to change your contributions.

Account Rollovers and Transfers

HSA-Rollover

If you have more than one HSA, maybe from a previous job or because you wanted to set up separate accounts with a specific administrator, you are allowed to make transfers between your HSAs. Money that is transferred between Health Savings Accounts doesn't count toward your contribution limit for the year, since it was already counted when it first went into your HSA.

When you transfer money from an old HSA into a new account, your old starting date is rolled over with it. This means that you have continual coverage starting from when you established your first HSA. This is important because you can only reimburse expenses incurred after your account was established. You'll want to make sure your account shows the earliest start date possible so more of your expenses can be paid from your HSA.

Money can be transferred directly from one HSA to another as long as both administrators allow it. If your administrator doesn't process direct transfers, you can withdraw money from one HSA and deposit it in another within 60 days with no penalty. If the money is not deposited within the 60-day window, it will need to be claimed on your income taxes and a 20% excise fee paid on any amount not used for qualified medical expenses.

You are always allowed to withdraw money from your HSA, but an administrator is not required to accept the transferred funds. Talk to your account administrator first to find out their transfer procedure. They may even be able to help you find an easier way to manage your accounts.

If you have an Archer MSA, an early version of an HSA that is no longer available, these same rules apply.

IRA Transfer

In addition to moving money between HSAs, you can also move money from your IRA into an HSA. This sort of transfer can only be done once in your lifetime, though, so use it wisely. You can only transfer money from a traditional IRA or a Roth IRA, not from a 401(k), SEP, or other retirement plan. Money that is transferred from an IRA to an HSA does count toward your contribution limit for the year.

The one exception to the once-in-a-lifetime rule is that if you make a contribution from your IRA to reach your individual limit for the year and then get married or have a child and switch to a family plan, you can make a second contribution up to the family limit as long as both transfers happen in the same calendar year.

A 12-consecutive-month testing period starts the month that you transfer funds from an IRA to an HSA. If you lose eligibility at any point during those 12 months, you will need to count the transferred funds on your tax return as part of your income and pay a 10% excise tax.

> Transferring money from a regular savings account is considered a regular contribution. You cannot move money from an FSA or an HRA into your HSA.

Excess Contributions

In case you do go over your contribution limit for the year, you should work with your administrator to remove any excess as soon as possible. Any extra money that remains in your HSA past your tax deadline (usually April 15th of the following calendar year) will be subject to a 6% excise tax. Money contributed in excess needs to be withdrawn along with whatever earnings was gained on that amount through interest or investments. You will also need to include that amount in your gross income for the year. You will still pay regular income tax on the money, but if you can withdraw the money before the tax deadline you can avoid the penalty tax.

To calculate earnings made on your excess contributions, use the following:

$$\text{Net Income} = \frac{\text{Contribution} \times (\text{Closing Balance} - \text{Opening Balance})}{\text{Opening Balance}}$$

Your opening balance is the amount in your HSA once you make the contribution, and your closing balance is the amount in your HSA just before you receive your contribution back, with adjustments made for any additional contributions or withdrawals.

Contribution Example 4

On May 1, 2018, when Alicia's HSA is worth $4,800, she makes a $1,600 contribution to her HSA. She then requests that $400 of the contribution be returned to her as an excess contribution. On February 1, 2019, when the HSA is worth $7,600, her HSA trustee distributes the $400 plus attributable net income. During this time, no other contributions or distributions have been made.

The adjusted opening balance is $6,400 ($4,800 + $1,600), and the adjusted closing balance is $7,600. So the calculation for Alicia's net income is 400 x (7,600 − 6,400) / 6,400, or $75. This results in a total distribution of $475. The $400 is not subject to the penalty tax, but the $75 of net income is.

You can only withdraw excess funds in the case of an accidental over-contribution, and only up until the tax filing deadline. After the deadline has passed, you still need to withdraw the money, but you will be subject to the excise tax for each year that the extra money was in the account. Rules on how to withdraw extra funds are different between administrators, so contact your administrator to make sure that they are aware of your withdrawal and that it is reported correctly.

Chapter 3: Distributions

Qualified Expenses

Once you establish an HSA and are contributing to it, you can start making distributions for qualified medical expenses, like:
- Prescription medications
- Doctor visits
- Eyeglasses and examination fees
- Dental care
- Hospital bills

Generally, anything that is not covered by your insurance or other coverage and is considered a medical necessity can be paid with money from your HSA. These are defined by tax law and include expenses for the diagnosis, cure, mitigation, treatment, or prevention of disease. This applies to your doctor visits and prescriptions, but it also includes some items that might surprise you.

Expense	Explanation
Guide Dog or Service Animal	Your HSA money can help pay for a service animal if you have a physical disability, both for helping you to get the animal and to pay for ongoing care.
Home Improvement	Classified as a capital expense, if you make changes to your home or install special equipment designed to help you take care of yourself or one of your dependents you can pay part of the expense with HSA dollars.

Insurance Premiums	You can't pay for your regular premiums with HSA dollars, but you can use HSA funds if you are collecting unemployment, are on COBRA continuing coverage, or are paying for long-term insurance. Some Medicare premiums are also able to be paid from your HSA.
Nursing Home	So long as the main reason for someone to be in the nursing home is for medical care, the costs for lodging and meals all count as eligible expenses.
Special Education	If a doctor recommends that a child receive special education from a particular tutor or school, the cost of receiving that care can be paid for with your HSA. This is primarily designed to provide tools for children with a disability, like learning braille or sign language.
Transportation Expenses	A standard mileage rate, a set limit for hotel rooms per night, and other travel expenses can be reimbursed from your HSA if you need to travel to a specific doctor to receive medical care.

While these might be considered qualified medical expenses that can be paid using money from your HSA, they often don't count toward your deductible for the year. Only things that might be covered by medical insurance will count toward your deductible.

In addition to paying for your qualified medical expenses, you can also use your HSA to reimburse qualified expenses for your spouse and any dependents you can claim on your taxes. This is true even if that person isn't eligible for their own HSA. Federal guidelines on dependents are listed under the Internal Revenue Code (IRC), Section 152.

A longer list of qualified medical expenses is included in the appendix. For a full list of covered expenses, visit the IRS website at

www.irs.gov/forms-instructions and search for Publication 502 on Medical and Dental Expenses, released annually.

The Distribution Process

How you manage your distributions will be largely based on your administrator. Many administrators will provide you with a debit card or checks that you can use to make payments directly from your HSA.

You can also request reimbursement by check or a deposit directly to your account. This is useful if you are unable to use your card or need to reimburse an expense at a later date. Keep track of your withdrawals so you can properly report your eligible expenses when you file your tax return.

Administrators are allowed to put some restrictions on disbursements, like limiting the number of withdrawals per month or establishing a minimum amount of money you can withdraw at one time. Be sure to find out what those restrictions might be for you. While there might be some reasonable restrictions in place on amounts and frequency of withdrawal, the money in your HSA is still yours, and you can use it as needed.

Save Receipts

You do not need to submit a receipt to withdraw funds from your account or pay for your medical expenses, but it is still important to keep track of your expenses and hold onto your receipts in case of an IRS audit. If you have a Health FSA or HRA, you may already be in the habit of saving all your medical receipts and Explanations of Benefits (EOBs). You'll want to keep in those same habits or start building them up for your HSA.

Many HSAs will come with debit cards that are pre-programmed to only pay for medical expenses, either at the store or the doctor's office. For these purchases, information about what you bought including where and when you bought it is automatically sent back to your HSA. This information is then stored and can be used as needed without you needing to scan and send in a receipt. For these purchases, keeping your receipts merely allows you to check that the information is correct and create your own personal records.

You won't always be able to pay your medical expenses with your debit card, perhaps because your administrator doesn't provide one or the person you are paying doesn't accept your card. Keep records of all these unpaid expenses. Your receipts and EOBs will let you validate your purchases and help you keep track of amounts when you reimburse yourself later.

Another reason to hold onto your receipts is that you can reimburse yourself for any expense incurred after your HSA was established, even if you weren't eligible to contribute. You can even reimburse yourself for expenses that are years old, getting the money in one lump sum, all tax free. To do this, you'll need to have your receipts in order so you know exactly how much you can take out as a qualified medical expense. Make sure you have enough evidence to prove that you really did incur the expense and that you were the person who paid for it, rather than your insurance or other coverage stepping in and paying the bill.

While it is ultimately your job to keep track of your expenses and reimbursements, a full service HSA administrator can help with the record-keeping process. The IRS requires that receipts and other evidence of qualified medical expenses be kept as far back as seven years in case of an audit. Keeping track of that much documentation can be exhausting, so it's useful to have an administrator that helps you to upload and store receipts for the future.

Fees on Non-Eligible Withdrawals

While you are allowed to use your money however you see fit, there are some penalties on using it on anything other than a qualified medical expense. So if you decide to withdraw a thousand dollars to go on a nice cruise, no matter how beneficial that might be to your wellbeing, it won't count as a qualified expense. That amount will need to be reported as part of your income for the year, and you'll pay both taxes and an additional excise tax. Currently, the excise tax is at 20% of the withdrawn amount.

You may also be subject to the excise fee if you withdraw money from one HSA in order to transfer that amount to another account but fail to deposit it within 60 days of the withdrawal. Once you have passed your 60 day deadline to deposit that money, the amount must be reported as income and the excise fee paid.

Once you turn 65, the excise fee no longer applies. You can withdraw the money you need to take your cruise and only pay income taxes on the amount. The same is true if you become disabled. Of course, when you use your money for qualified medical expenses even the income tax doesn't apply.

Another option you have to access your money is to delay reimbursement. Your expenses can be reimbursed to you at any time, even years into the future, as long as you never closed your HSA and can validate the expense. If you keep track of your records and your account, you can pay your medical expenses out-of-pocket and use your saved receipts to reimburse those expenses all at once with tax-free dollars. This lets you access your money tax-free when you need it and lets it stay in your account and grow as long as possible with interest and investments.

Chapter 4: Account Management

Establishing Your HSA

One of the big decisions you'll need to make in establishing your HSA is choosing a full-service administrator or other IRS-approved custodian and working with them to set up your account. Your HSA-eligible health plan may come with a recommended administrator or automatically set you up with one particular company. You can choose to work with that administrator or to open your own account with a different provider and transfer funds to that HSA.

Any entity that has been approved by the IRS to administer IRAs is automatically approved to administer HSAs, plus any company that meets IRS standards to become an HSA administrator. This includes entities like national banks or brokerage houses as well as your local bank or credit union, as well as companies that are specifically designed for administering retirement accounts.

There are four main areas in which an administrator needs to provide services for accountholders, and it is important to choose one that matches your needs.

> **Contribution Management** – ability to receive contributions through a variety of methods, including electronically, in person, and by mail
> **Investment Management** – offers a variety of choices, fees, and flexibility for investing in different types of accounts
> **Withdrawal Management** – provides multiple methods for making withdrawals from the account for eligible expenses, including issuing a debit card and providing reimbursements

Record Keeping – processes enrollment; verifies eligibility; tracks contribution limits; liaisons with insurance companies, employers, and custodians; maintains account balance; receives and records all receipts; issues appropriate year-end tax forms

No matter who you decide to establish your HSA with, you'll want to make sure you have a clear understanding of their fees, withdrawal and reimbursement guidelines, investing options, and any extra services they can provide for you.

It's a good idea to get everything ready to establish your HSA ahead of time so you can make your initial deposit as soon as you are eligible. You can only use your HSA for expenses incurred after your account is established, so you want to get the earliest start date possible.

Invest your Savings

Your HSA works in two ways: helping you to pay for qualified medical expenses now and helping you to save money for your expenses in retirement.

It's important to save for your medical expenses post-retirement, since they will count as a major component of your post-retirement finances. According to a recent report, a couple retiring in 2017 and living for 20 years in retirement might expect to pay $275,000 in insurance premiums.[v] That level of savings can be hard to build up on your own. This is where your HSA steps in to help.

Always remember that your HSA money doesn't just go in tax-free and come out tax-free for qualified expenses. It also grows tax-free with interest, dividends, and other investment gains. Like with any other account, the more money you have saved the more it will be able to grow. Because of this, it's important to contribute all the way up to your yearly limit if possible and invest as much of that money as you can.

Investing your HSA money will give your account the potential for higher return than saving alone. There is some risk involved with investments, and money you've invested is harder to access than money in savings, but the opportunity for growth available with investments will help your account keep up with inflation and cover expenses into retirement.

Your investment options will vary depending on your administrator. Some administrators provide a direct link for you to invest your HSA money with a major investment company and a way to transfer money between your benefit account and the investment account. Other administrators provide a variety of investment options for you to choose from. You can often specify how much money you want to be invested in each product.

It's a good idea to keep some money in savings so you can reimburse current medical expenses and avoid liquidating your investments prematurely. Think ahead for big expenses and try to have the necessary money available as you need it. Anything that you don't need available in savings you can invest to maximize your growth potential. You can also choose to pay all of your qualified expenses out-of-pocket and reimburse yourself later once your investments have matured.

It's a good idea to start an HSA while you are younger and healthier. The earlier you start building your account, the longer it has time to grow and the more of an impact it will have in retirement. It also helps you to build good habits for your health and finances from a young age.

Investing Example

Aaron, Bridget, and Casey all decide to switch from a traditional health plan to an HSA-eligible health plan. They all will save $100 a month on the lower premium, and all three expect to spend about $1,000 a year on medical expenses.

Aaron chooses to contribute the $100 a month that he saves on his premiums into his HSA. He saves money with his tax-free contributions, and he has money set aside for the medical expenses he has throughout the year. He pays for expenses as he goes, and at the end of the year he still has $200 in his HSA.

Bridget also chooses to put in the $100 a month she saves on premiums, but she decides not to reimburse her expenses right away. Instead, she pays for her qualified medical expenses out of pocket and saves her receipts so that she can grow her account faster. At the end of the first year, she has $1,200 in her HSA. Once she reaches $2,000 in her account, she can start investing her account. The investments grow tax free, and, when she needs some extra money, she can go back and reimburse some of her old expenses while keeping her HSA healthy for when she retires.

Casey chooses to contribute the maximum amount every year and not reimburse any expenses right away. She can start investing her money right away, and with more money to invest it can grow more. She also can reimburse her expenses when she needs to, and she is able to set aside more money for retirement.

At the end of ten years, Aaron will have accumulated $2,000 plus whatever he earned in interest. Bridget will have accumulated $12,000, minus what she reimbursed herself for and plus what she earned through investments. Casey will have accumulated more than $35,000, minus her expenses and plus what she earned by investing.

Fund HSA First

If you have multiple types of savings accounts for your medical expenses or retirement funds, you should focus on contributing to your HSA before your other accounts. An HSA has advantages over other accounts that make it better to fully fund this account before any others.

If you have an HSA and a Limited Purpose FSA that covers your dental or vision care, contribute all the way up to your HSA before contributing to your LPFSA. The money in an HSA can be used for all the same expenses as an LPFSA and also won't expire at the end of the year. Once you've reached your contribution limit for an HSA, you should find out exactly how much you expect to pay from your LPFSA and only contribute that amount so you aren't losing money at the end of the year. An LPFSA is a way for you to avoid spending your HSA dollars while still getting a tax benefit, so it is a good idea to contribute to an LPFSA if possible, but only after you've fully funded your HSA.

Only an HSA is tax-free or tax-deductible on both contributions and eligible distributions, so if you have an IRA, Roth IRA, or other retirement account in addition to your HSA, you still may want to contribute to your HSA first. The money in a traditional IRA is contributed tax-free but is taxed for any distributions. The money in a Roth IRA is distributed tax-free, but your contributions are taxed. Your HSA money is both contributed and distributed with a tax advantage.

HSAs do have an excise fee on non-eligible distributions, but that fee is waived after you turn 65 or qualify for disability. Retirement accounts are only accessible after you turn $59\frac{1}{2}$, retire, or start receiving disability benefits. But since an HSA does let you access your money early if necessary and gives you tax-free distributions on qualified medical expenses, your funds are still available earlier with an HSA than with a retirement account. An HSA also doesn't have any forced withdrawals, while an IRA starts requiring you to withdraw funds by April 1st the year after you turn $70\frac{1}{2}$.

You may want to fund your IRA or other retirement fund over your HSA if your IRA provides a significant advantage in investment options. Even if this is the case, you can always open a different HSA where you have access to the investments you need and transfer your money to that account. Legally, the investment options between IRAs and HSAs are the same—you just need to find an administrator who will give you the variety that you need.

Tips on Saving

Once you have established your HSA, you will want to make sure you are using your money wisely and taking advantage of all available options to save money. Here are some things you can do to save.

Take Advantage of Preventive Care

Under the Affordable Care Act, all plans are required to cover preventive care. This usually includes regular doctor appointments, vaccines for children, wellness programs, and women's care. Find out what your plan covers and take advantage of those benefits as much as possible.

Stay in Network

Just like a traditional health plan, your HSA-eligible health plan will be part of a network of preferred providers. Those are the doctors and hospitals that your plan has contracted with to provide you services at agreed prices. For example, your plan may have worked with its in-network doctors to determine that $150 is the correct amount for you to pay for an x-ray. If you choose to go out of network, you may be charged more.

In addition, only the agreed-upon amount will count toward your in-network deductible. Anything spent beyond that will only count toward your out-of-network expenses, which can be higher than the IRS deductible limit. If you rely heavily on out-of-network care, you could end up paying more than your deductible each year before your co-insurance starts.

Look for Discounts

Being on an HSA-eligible health plan means you can't be a part of any program that offers you reimbursements for your medical expenses. However, you are allowed to receive discounts on expenses like your prescriptions. Since this qualifies as a change in prices and not reimbursement, you can still count this cost toward your deductible and pay for it with your HSA while remaining eligible to contribute.

You should also always ask about generic options for your prescriptions. These will cost less and help you to save money.

Choose Your Care Wisely

Not every sniffle needs a trip to the doctor, but going in to get treatment for that lingering cough can help you avoid getting stuck in the hospital due to a bad case of pneumonia. Know your body, and make the decision that is most sensible for your health and for your savings account. That doesn't mean not going to the emergency room when you do have an emergency, but it might mean taking a few days off work and getting lots of rest instead of going to the doctor for your head cold.

Tax Reporting

When it actually comes time to file your taxes, it can be hard knowing exactly how to record your HSA contributions and withdrawals. Just because money is contributed to and withdrawn from your HSA tax-free doesn't mean that the IRS doesn't want to know about it. The rules on reporting can be complex, and we recommend speaking to your tax advisor or accountant to make sure that you are getting everything right for your specific scenario. If you are doing your tax preparations by yourself, though, here's what you need to know.

You can't get a deduction twice.

If your HSA contributions were made pre-tax directly out of your paycheck or through an employer contribution, you can't count them as an above-the-line item on your tax return to get the deduction taken again. If you paid for a qualified medical expense out of your HSA, you can't take a deduction on that same expense, since that money has already been deducted from your taxes. In short, you can't double-dip on tax deductions.

You get all deductions on your HSA

No matter who made the contribution to your HSA – you, your employer, your friends and family – you get the deduction. Similarly, if you made a contribution to someone else's HSA, that person gets the tax deduction rather than you. Any contributions made post-tax, whether from you or someone else, should be taken as a line-item deduction on your tax return.

Reporting non-eligible withdrawals

If you did need to withdraw money for a non-eligible expense, that money needs to be included in your taxable income for the year. In addition, if you are under the age of 65 and not on disability, you will need to pay an additional 20% excise tax on the amount withdrawn.

Over-contributions

If you aren't able to withdraw the extra money from your HSA, you'll need to report the extra money contributed as part of your income and pay an additional 6% tax on the extra. Your deadline to work with your administrator to withdraw the excess is tax day (usually April 15th) the year following your over-contribution.

When reporting your HSA withdrawals and contributions, you'll need to complete Form 8889. That information will then transfer onto your 1040 form. You should receive a form 1099-SA from your HSA administrator, which will give you information on all the withdrawals for the year. Your W-2 that you receive from your employer will automatically report all of your pre-tax contributions under Box 12, code W so that they are already separated from your post-tax contributions.

Any contributions that you or anyone else make to your account post-tax will be reported on a form 5498-SA that your administrator will send to you. This amount is deductible on your tax return.

Expenses that are not paid by your health insurance, employer health plan, or reimbursed from your HSA can be included in your normal itemized deductions, but if you do take a deduction on that amount you cannot reimburse yourself for the expense at a later point in time.

Remember, it is your responsibility to accurately report your contributions and withdrawals to the IRS, including knowing when you have gone over your contribution limits and when you have withdrawn money for non-qualified expenses. Keep track of your account so that you can be ready to report.

Chapter 5: What about...?

Medicare

Medicare is a medical program available to people age 65 and older or to people who have been on Social Security Disability Income (SSDI) for 24 consecutive months. Many people choose to enroll in social security benefits once they turn 65, which automatically enrolls them in Medicare Part A. Being enrolled in any Medicare coverage automatically disqualifies you from being eligible to establish or contribute to an HSA.

However, even if you do enroll in Medicare, you can still use the HSA money you have already contributed to pay for your Medicare premiums and for any other qualified medical expenses that come up without being subject to income tax. You can also choose not to enroll in Medicare when you turn 65 in order to continue contributing to your HSA.

In addition to using your HSA funds for medical expenses, you can also begin to take money out of your account for other expenses without paying the 20% excise fee once you turn 65. Just remember that the amount you have withdrawn from your HSA must be noted as income for the year and taxes must be paid on anything not used for qualified expenses.

FMLA

If you are on leave under the Family and Medical Leave Act (FMLA), you can maintain your HSA eligibility as long as you maintain your health coverage. Your employer will still cover whatever portion of premiums is normally covered and require that you pay the rest either out of whatever pay you are still receiving or out-of-pocket. If you choose not to continue your health coverage, you will no longer be eligible to contribute to your HSA.

Continuing Coverage

The Consolidated Omnibus Budget Reconciliation Act of 1985 (COBRA) requires employers with 20 or more employees to allow those employees to continue their benefits coverage when their job ends or there is a reduction of hours. You can keep the exact same benefits that you had under your former position, but you will pay the full amount of the premium instead of your employer picking up any portion of the bill. As long as you are still covered under your HSA-eligible health plan, you can continue contributing to your HSA, though your contributions will now be made after tax.

While the expense on premiums does mean that you are paying more every month, a high-deductible health plan will often have lower premiums than a traditional health plan. Choosing to continue your health plan through COBRA can allow you to keep your coverage consistent while you are transitioning between jobs. The expense may also be worth it, since it can help you to keep coverage until the end of a testing period so you don't have to pay fees or back-taxes on over-contributions. You can also use your HSA dollars to pay for your COBRA premiums, lessening the impact of those costs.

Losing and Regaining Eligibility

Your eligibility affects whether you can start or contribute to an HSA each month, but once you have established an HSA you can always withdraw funds from it. So even if you lose your eligibility to contribute by switching jobs, retiring, or some other reason, you can still spend your HSA dollars and should keep track of your account. If you run out of money in your HSA, that account is closed. You will have to start over with a new account if you become eligible again. Any expenses during the time you didn't have an HSA can't be reimbursed by your new account.

Remember that monthly fees that come directly out of your HSA will also affect the balance. Because of this, you might want to consider keeping some of your money in an HSA that doesn't have any monthly fees or looking for an administrator that will let you pay the fees directly instead of withdrawing them from the account. This way you can keep that money set aside in order to keep your HSA open if you do unexpectedly lose eligibility. You can always go back later and reimburse your expenses once you have eligibility again, but once your HSA is closed that opportunity is gone.

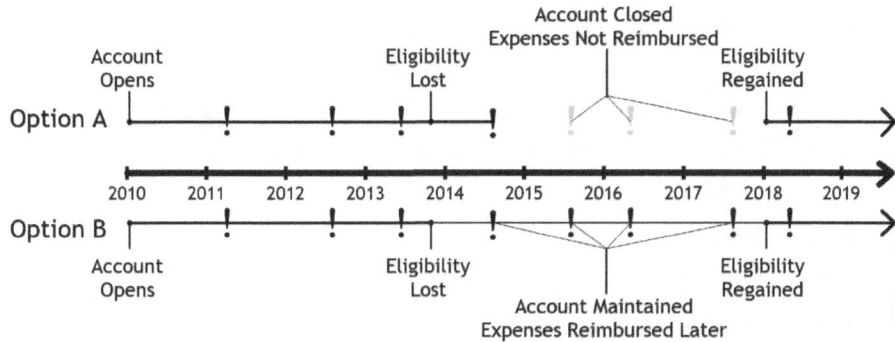

Even if you aren't planning on keeping a balance in your HSA in case of later eligibility, you will still need to track your expenses so you can report your withdrawals to the IRS and have documentation in case of an audit. You'll also want to track how much money you have left in your account so you know how much can be reimbursed.

> ### Maintaining Your Account Example
> Avery established her first Health Savings Account on her very first day of eligibility, February 1, 2010. In 2013, she lost her job and HSA-eligible plan but still had a few thousand dollars in her HSA. She used some of the money for minor expenses but put most of it into investments.
>
> In August of 2014, Avery fell and broke her arm. She knew she still had money in her HSA she could use to pay for the medical bill, but she also knew that if she chose to use that money, her HSA would close and she'd have to start over again with a new account if she ever regained eligibility.

Instead of using her HSA money for her broken arm, Avery paid for her medical expenses out-of-pocket and kept all the receipts and EOBs from the doctors. When she switched jobs again in 2018, her new employer had an HSA-eligible plan option. Avery was able to start a new HSA and move all her remaining money from her old account so she has continuous coverage starting back in February 2010.

Once Avery had contributed more money to her HSA, she submitted all the receipts and EOBs she saved from her broken arm. Because she kept a balance in her old account, she can also reimburse any other qualified medical expenses from the time when she wasn't eligible to contribute. The money that stayed in her HSA also grew from investments so that she has even more money for future expenses.

TRICARE and IHS Coverage

If you are eligible for TRICARE or Indian Health Service (IHS) coverage, you can still be eligible for an HSA as long as you have not received medical services through these providers for at least 3 months. Receiving dental, vision, or preventive care with any of these providers does not affect your HSA eligibility.

If you do receive medical (disqualifying) treatment through TRICARE or IHS, you are ineligible to contribute to an HSA for the next three months from receiving care. For example, if you visit a doctor on March 3rd, you will be ineligible for April, May, and June. You will need to prorate your contribution limit for the year to account for any months you were ineligible.

Receiving service for a service-connected disability at a VA hospital will not impact HSA eligibility. A service-connected disability is a disability received in the line of duty while in the active military, naval, or air service. This only applies to coverage under VA programs, not to TRICARE.

Divorce

Each HSA is owned by just one person, and the money that is in it belongs to that person. This generally means that in the case of a divorce, each person keeps their HSA and those funds. Interest earned in an HSA can be transferred under a divorce or separation agreement.

Children of divorced parents are considered eligible dependents of both parents. Either parent can reimburse medical expenses for that child, though the same expense cannot be claimed by both parents.

Death

Your HSA is part of your assets, and like anything else you own it will be passed on to your beneficiary as you have directed. If the account goes to your spouse, it automatically becomes their HSA, and they can use it just like a regular HSA. If the account is passed on to someone other than your spouse, they can still be reimbursed up to a year later for any qualified medical expenses that you accrued up until your death. Any remaining money after that will be liquidated and count as part of their taxable income for the year. If you don't have a beneficiary, the account is liquidated and counted as part of your estate.

State Rules

Your state may have some specific rules regarding HSAs. For example, even though there is no federal tax on HSA contributions, some states, like Alabama, Wisconsin, New Jersey, and California, do assess tax. Many states also have specific rules defining tax dependents that may impact which of your dependents' expenses you are able to reimburse. Your account start date can also be affected by state law. This is impacted by where your HSA administrator is located, not necessarily where you live.

Your best resources for finding out what rules apply to you are your tax advisor or HSA administrator.

Conclusion: Is HSA Right for You?

Taking Control of Your Health

Some people feel that an HSA-eligible health plan is only good for people who are in good health and have a lot of disposable income—the "healthy and wealthy." While people who are able to max out their contributions will receive the full tax benefits on their HSA savings, the tax benefits and lower premiums still help people who aren't able to contribute the full amount. And while you won't have as many medical expenses if you are healthy, this is true no matter what plan you have. Someone who goes to the doctor frequently but is careful to stay in network and check prescription costs may find that an HSA-eligible plan actually saves money over a traditional plan.

The key traits that will help an HSA-eligible plan work are not "healthy and wealthy" but "careful and wise." If you are paying attention to your expenses and weighing the benefits and risks of your different options, you can find out where and how to save money with an HSA. Once you can see the opportunities to save, you can see if making the switch is right for you.

Your first step in taking ownership of your healthcare spending is deciding if an HSA-eligible plan is the right option for you. A side-by-side comparison can help you to see how much you might expect to spend with each type of plan.

Start by determining what medical expenses you expect to see in the next year. You can use your past year's expenses as a guide, but keep in mind any big family changes you're expecting, like getting married or having a new baby.

Once you have an idea of what expenses you are expecting, take a look at your different health coverage options to see which plan will save you the most money. There are even online calculators that can help you to compare your traditional health plan to an HSA-eligible HDHP.

Plan Comparison Example 1

Angela just turned 26 and is losing coverage under her parents. She is selecting her own health insurance through work, which offers both a traditional health plan and an HSA-eligible health plan.

The traditional plan will cost her $1,500 a year in premiums, and the HSA-eligible plan will cost $1,050 in premiums. Additionally, her employer is offering $300 in HSA contributions to any full-time employee who signs up.

Last year, Angela only went to the doctor twice, once for her yearly check-up and once for a prescription when she got strep throat. Under her parents' traditional plan, she paid a $20 copay and $10 for the prescription. She estimates that her expenses for the coming year will be similar, meaning that under a traditional plan she will spend about $1,530 on premiums and medical expenses for the year.

Looking up costs for the doctor's visits, Angela learns that it will cost $120 to go to the doctor under an HSA-eligible plan, and the same strep throat medicine she got last time would cost $180. However, a generic version of the same prescription would only cost $40, and with her yearly checkup being covered under preventive care, she estimates her expenses under an HSA-eligible plan to be about $1,210 for the year.

Angela decides to go with the HSA option and contribute an extra $500 to her account in addition to the $300 offered by her employer. She expects to spend about $200 of that on medical care, which would leave $600 in her HSA to roll over for the next year. Overall, she's put aside $1,550 for her healthcare expenses – about the same as she would have spent under a traditional plan – and still has $600 in her HSA at the end of the year for future expenses.

Plan Comparison Example 2

The Barnes family is considering switching from a traditional health plan to an HSA-eligible HDHP. They have two young children, and last year they took 4 trips to the doctor and needed 5 different prescriptions, most of them antibiotics. Mr. Barnes also has asthma medicine that he takes regularly.

The traditional health plan option charges $4,500 in premiums, and the HSA-eligible option is being offered for $3,150. Mr. Barnes' employer is also offering $500 in HSA contributions for employees with family coverage.

Last year the family spent $80 in copays and $80 in prescription costs, with $60 of that being toward Mr. Barnes' asthma medicine. With the same estimated costs for next year, they expect to pay $4,660 under a traditional plan.

Under an HSA-eligible HDHP, the family would pay $120 per doctor's visit, for a total of $480 for 4 visits. They also would spend an estimated $560 on prescriptions. But with a lower premium, they expect that total expenses for the year under an HSA-eligible plan would come to only $4,190.

By choosing the HSA option and putting aside an extra $1,500 into an HSA, the Barnes' family puts a total $4,650 towards their healthcare. That's slightly less than their expected expenses under a traditional plan. With the additional $500 in employer contributions, they can pay for all medical expenses out of their HSA and still have $960 in their HSA to use for the next year.

> *Plan Comparison Example 3*
>
> Corey currently pays $2,500 a year in premiums for a traditional health plan that covers himself and his son. Corey's workplace has just started offering an HSA-eligible health plan with family coverage starting at $2,000 for the year.
>
> Corey and his son are both diabetic and require regular insulin shots and testing supplies. Under their current plan, they spend about $1,000 a year on medical supplies. Corey estimates that under an HSA-eligible plan, they will spend all the way up to the $5,000 deductible limit due to insulin costs.
>
> While switching to an HSA-eligible plan might help Corey to save money on premiums, that doesn't balance out the higher amount he would need to spend on prescriptions. He chooses to stay with his traditional plan.

The most important thing to remember when you are under an HSA-eligible plan is that it is a consumer-driven plan. Therefore, you are responsible for your healthcare. It's up to you to know your eligibility status, your contribution limits, your eligible expenses, and your account balance. Your administrator will be able to help you with tracking your expenses and your account, but the ultimate responsibility for your healthcare is up to you.

Appendix I: Qualified Medical Expenses

This list is not complete. For a more complete list of tax-deductible expenses, review IRS Publication 502, which is released annually. Items that are for medical use only generally do not require a doctor's note to justify reimbursement, but most medicines and other dual-purpose items will require some form of professional recommendation to justify the expense in case of an audit.

Please note that not all items listed in Publication 502 are eligible for HSA reimbursement, as certain items are not listed on the subset list of HSA qualified expenses. Please review IRS Code §213(d) for more information on qualified expenses and dependents. All expenses should be primarily for medical care and are subject to IRS review and approval.

- **Abortion** – legal procedures only
- **Artificial Limbs**
- **Bandages and First Aid Supplies**
- **Birth Control Pills**
- **Capital Expenses** – includes the amount paid to install special equipment if the main purpose is medical care. The eligible cost is reduced by the value of improvement to your property. Amount paid for upkeep of a capital asset can also qualify.
- **Dental Treatment**
- **Diagnostic Devices** – includes items like thermometers and blood sugar test kits
- **Eye Care** – includes contacts, glasses, exams, and surgery
- **Guide Dog or other Service Animal**
- **Hearing Aids**

- **Insurance Premiums** – only applies if under COBRA, collecting unemployment, or for qualified long-term care insurance. For individuals over 65, includes Medicare A or B or other premiums. Only covers medical portion of any insurance. Contact your tax advisor or HSA administrator for more details, or review IRS Publication 502.
- **Lead-Based Paint Removal** – if paint is accessible to child with lead poisoning
- **Lifetime Care-Advanced Payments** – includes payments to retirement home under promise for lifetime care including medical care; also referred to as "founders fee." Also includes payments to ensure care of disabled dependent after parent's death.
- **Long-Term Care** – includes premiums and cost of care for all medical expenses for someone who is chronically ill and receiving care on the recommendation of a doctor. These contracts are only eligible under specific criteria and only up to a set limit on premiums.
- **Medical Information Plan** – includes payments to keep medical information to provide to doctors upon request
- **Medical Treatment** – includes physical exams, tests, lab fees, hospital services, inpatient and outpatient care, operations/surgery, transplants
- **Medicines** – must be prescribed by a doctor, except for insulin
- **Mental healthcare** – includes psychiatric care, psychoanalysis, psychologist, therapy
- **Nursing Home** – includes all expenses if primary reason for being in the home is medical
- **Nursing Services** – do not have to be provided by a certified nurse but can only cover cost of medical services, not household or personal services
- **Pregnancy Test Kit**
- **Reconstructive Surgery**

- **Recovery Programs** – includes alcohol, drug addiction, smoking, and weight-loss
- **Special Education** – must be doctor-recommended for a child working to overcome a disability
- **Specialist Care** – includes acupuncture, Christian Science practitioner, osteopath
- **Technology** – includes cost to install special equipment or the price difference between normal technology and specialized technology for cars, telephones, and televisions
- **Travel Expenses** – if traveling for medical treatment, includes cost of travel and lodging up to set amount.

Glossary

- **Health Savings Account (HSA)** – an individual savings account for you to put aside money tax-free to use for qualified medical expenses now or in the future
- **High-Deductible Health Plan (HDHP)** – a health plan that differs from a traditional health plan by having a higher deductible and lower premiums; having coverage under an HSA-eligible HDHP is the only way to open and contribute to an HSA
- **Deductible** – the amount of money you pay to a provider before your insurance or other medical coverage starts to kick in a percentage of the cost; expenses you pay for medical care, prescriptions, and certain premiums all count toward your deductible
- **Out-of-pocket Maximum** – the maximum amount you pay for covered services in a plan year. Once you have spent up to this amount on deductibles, copayments, and coinsurance, your health plan pays 100% of the cost of covered benefits. Your out-of-pocket limit doesn't include monthly premiums.
- **Premium** – the amount spent for coverage in your health insurance or employer health plan
- **Coinsurance** – the amount of an expense, usually a percentage, that you are still responsible for paying once meeting your deductible
- **Dependent** – for health coverage, can include children up to age 26 and spouses. For reimbursing medical expenses from your HSA, is limited to qualified children or other relatives who can be claimed as dependents on your taxes. The requirements on dependents are outlined by the Internal Revenue Code (IRC) Section 152.
- **Health Flexible Spending Accounts (Health FSAs)** – similar to HSAs in allowing you to set aside pre-tax dollars for medical costs, but these accounts don't invest and are "use-it-or-lose-it" accounts that reset back to $0 at the start of the new year;

can include grace or carryover period allowing amounts to carry a few months into the next year
- **Health Reimbursement Arrangements (HRAs)** – a Health Savings Account funded entirely through employer contributions; not portable
- **Limited Plan Flexible Spending Account (LPFSA)** – an FSA designed to work with an HSA that might only cover dental, vision, and/or preventive expenses or, more rarely, only cover expenses after a deductible is met
- **Cafeteria Plan** – a style of benefit coverage that allows employees to make pre-tax deductions for selected benefits including health coverage
- **Medical Savings Accounts (MSAs)** – also known as Archer's Medical Savings Accounts or Archer MSAs. MSAs were originally introduced in 1996 as the first version of the Health Savings Account, which was only available to small businesses or self-employed individuals. When the 2003 bill expanded the role of HSAs, they were rebranded as Archer MSAs, and anyone who still had one could still use the money available but no new accounts could be opened.

Resources

The legal allowance for HSAs is detailed in IRC Section 223 on Health Savings Accounts. The IRS has also released several notices about HSA guidance as well as including information on HSAs in their yearly 969 publication. Other useful publications and notices include IRS Publication 502, which details eligible medical and dental expenses and IRS notices regarding HSA regulation.

You can access IRS forms, publications, and notices on their website at **www.irs.gov/forms-instructions**.

---

[i] OECD (2018), Health spending (indicator). doi: 10.1787/8643de7e-en (Accessed on 15 May 2018)

[ii] OECD (2018), Public spending on education (indicator). doi: 10.1787/f99b45d0-en (Accessed on 15 May 2018)

[iii] The World Bank. Military expenditure (% of GDP). Raw data. Stockholm International Peace Research Institute (SIPRI).

[iv] Devenir Research (2018), 2017 Year-End HSA Market Statistics & Trends Executive Summary. Devenir Group, LLC.

[v] Fidelity Viewpoints (2017), Retiree Health Care Costs Continue to Surge. September 6. https://www.fidelity.com/viewpoints/retirement/retiree-health-costs-rise.

About the Author

S.J. Klumpenhower is a certified HSA specialist and healthcare advisor with Erisa Trust Company. She is a professional writer and graduated summa cum laude from the University of New Mexico.

HSA: Start Here

Author / S.J. Klumpenhower
Publisher / EHGBooks United States
http://www.TaiwanFellowship.org
Date / July 2018
Distribution Channels
  Online
        Amazon.com
  China
        Xiamen International Book Company Limited
        Add: 4 / F, Logistics Building, No.8, Yuehua Road,
        Huli District, Xiamen City China
        Direct Line / 0592-5061658、6028707
  Taiwan & Hong Kong
        Sanmin Bookstores / http://www.sanmin.com.tw
        Add: No. 386, Fuxing N. Road, Taipei Taiwan
        Add: No. 61, Chongqing S. Road, Taipei Taiwan
        Direct Line / 02-2500-6600、02-2361-7511
        Kingstone Bookstores / http://www.kingstone.com.tw
Price / US$8 / NT$250 / RMB$55

2018 © United States, Permission required for reproduction, or translation in whole or part.

www.ingramcontent.com/pod-product-compliance
Lightning Source LLC
LaVergne TN
LVHW041544060526
838200LV00037B/1134